Hypertension

Information for this series, has been provided by Health Update, a monthly bulletin of the Society for Health Education and Learning Packages. The Update is intended to provide you with knowledge to adopt preventive measures and cooperate with the doctor during illness for better outcome of treatment.

Contributors

ALLOPATHY
Dr. S. Ramamurthy
(Assistant Professor, Department of Cardiology, All India Institute of Medical Sciences, New Delhi)

AYURVEDA
Dr. Rajni Sushma
(Senior Lecturer, A&U Tibbia Collage, New Delhi)

HOMOEOPATHY
Dr. V. K. Khanna
(Principal, Nehru Memorial Homoeopathic College, New Delhi)

NATURE CURE
Dr. Sambhashiva Rao
(Chief Medical Officer, Institute of Naturopathy, Bangalore)

Hypertension

Edited by
DR SAVITRI RAMAIAH

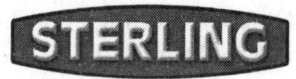

STERLING PAPERBACKS
An imprint of
Sterling Publishers (P) Ltd.
A-59, Okhla Industrial Area, Phase-II,
New Delhi-110020.
Tel: 26387070, 26386209; Fax: 91-11-26383788
E-mail: mail@sterlingpublishers.com
www.sterlingpublishers.com

Hypertension
© 2013, Sterling Publishers Private Limited
ISBN 978 81 207 8207 5

All rights are reserved.
No part of this publication may be reproduced, stored in a retrieval system or transmitted, in any form or by any means, mechanical, photocopying, recording or otherwise, without prior written permission of the original publisher.

Printed in India

Printed and Published by Sterling Publishers Pvt. Ltd., New Delhi-110 020.

Preface

Hypertension has been put together by *Health Update*, under the assistance of a team of medical experts who offer the latest perspectives on body health.

This book makes you an active participant in managing hypertension by giving multiple perspectives to choose from — allopathy, acupuncture, ayurveda, homoeopathy, nature cure and unani.

This book is intended as a home adviser but does not substitute a doctor.

The opinions are those of the contributors, and the publisher holds no responsibility.

Contents

Preface   5

Introduction   7

Allopathy   9

Ayurveda   53

Homoeopathy   59

Nature Cure   69

Definitions   77

References   79

Introduction

Hypertension or high blood pressure catches you unawares, in the prime of your life, as there are no symptoms. Stress, excessive salt, stiffening and thickening of the artery walls, increased retention of water and salt in the kidneys, obesity are some of the causes of hypertension.

Even mild hypertension can be risky. You can control hypertension by changing your lifestyle and by medicines. The management of diabetes, high cholesterol and smoking is important. Excessive intake of salt has to be curbed. Restriction of salt in diet is effective in about sixty percent of people with hypertension.

ALLOPATHY

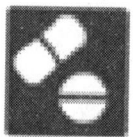

Hypertension is the term used for persistent high blood pressure. High blood pressure by itself is rarely fatal but, if not treated, can lead to serious complications. Prompt and proper management of hypertension reduces these complications.

What is blood pressure?

Every time your heart beats, it pumps out blood. This blood flows through three types of blood vessels: the *arteries*, the *capillaries* and the *veins* in that order, and returns to the heart again. The pressure resulting from the flow of blood in any of these vessels is called blood pressure (BP). When the doctor talks to you about blood pressure, he/she usually means the pressure of the flowing blood in the arteries.

A blood pressure reading has two numerical values: *"systolic"* and *"diastolic"*. When your heart contracts to force the blood out, the pressure in the arteries is maximum. This is called *"systolic pressure"*. At this time, the elastic walls of the large arteries are stretched. When your heart relaxes to be filled with blood from various parts of the body, the pressure in the arteries is minimum. This is called *"diastolic pressure"*. At this time, the elastic walls of the large arteries recoil. This recoil continues to push the blood forward against the resistance offered by the *arterioles*.

How is blood pressure recorded?

Blood pressure is usually measured in the artery of your arm using a *"sphygmomanometer"*. For many decades, blood pressure has been recorded in millimetres on a mercury column (mm of Hg). In recent times, sphygmomanometers without mercury columns (aneroid and digital instruments) are also used. They too express the readings as mm of Hg. *It is important to verify the readings from these instruments with a mercury sphygmomanometer regularly to ensure accuracy.*

A sphygmomanometer has an inflatable cuff which is wrapped around your arm. When the doctor pumps air into this cuff, the cuff exerts pressure on the soft tissues such as muscles and fat around the artery. This compresses the artery and the blood flow therefore stops. Gradual release of the air in the cuff results in partial opening of the artery causing a turbulent flow of blood. The point at which the blood begins to flow is heard by the doctor as distinct thumping sounds through a stethoscope placed over the artery. The reading on the sphygmomanometer at this point indicates your systolic pressure. Further gradual release of air from the cuff reduces pressure on the artery till it opens completely

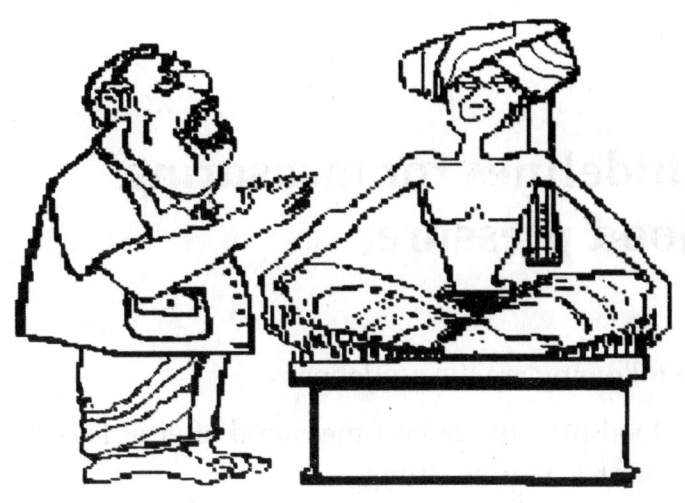

I am sure I will have a cure, but first tell me what is hypertension?

and the blood flows normally. The sounds of turbulent blood flow therefore disappear. The reading on the sphygmomanometer at this point denotes your diastolic pressure.

Numerical values of blood pressure are expressed as systolic pressure/diastolic pressure. If the doctor says that your blood pressure is 120/80, it means that your systolic pressure is 120 mm of Hg and your diastolic pressure is 80 mm of Hg.

Guidelines for measuring blood pressure

The following are the guidelines:
- Blood pressure is best measured after at least five minutes of quite sitting.
- Two readings three minutes apart are desirable, especially for those under stress.
- The cuff should be at the level of the smoking.
- Blood pressure should be measured at least one hour after taking meals or coffee.
- Blood pressure should not be measured within fifteen minutes of smoking.

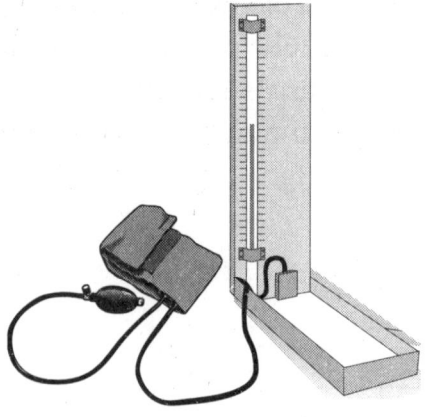

What are normal blood pressure values?

The normal adult systolic pressure ranges from 90-140 mm of Hg. The normal adult diastolic pressure ranges from 60-90 mm of Hg.

Blood pressure values are not constant throughout life. They are lower at birth and increase gradually with age. By the age of sixteen to eighteen years, blood pressure reaches adult levels. It is likely to increase further after the age of sixty years.

It is important to remember that your blood pressure changes from day to day and even from time to time on the same day. These variations are generally within normal limits and are observed mainly in the systolic pressure. Blood pressure is usually lower in the early mornings and higher in the late evenings. Physical exercise and emotional stress increase the blood pressure.

How are sudden changes in the blood pressure corrected?

The *vasomotor centre* of the brain corrects the sudden changes in your blood pressure without your knowledge. This is done by adjusting the peripheral resistance and/or cardiac output. Change in either of these two factors modifies the blood pressure because *blood pressure is the product of* **cardiac output** *and* **peripheral resistance.** Whenever the blood pressure rises, the vasomotor centre sends messages to the arterioles to relax. The peripheral resistance decreases and the blood pressure reaches normal levels. Similarly, when the blood pressure falls, the vasomotor centre sends messages to the arterioles to contract. Thus the peripheral resistance increases. The vasomotor centre also increases the cardiac output by increasing the activity of the heart. The combination of increased peripheral resistance and cardiac output increases the blood pressure and it reaches normal levels. The mechanism for correcting the sudden variations in blood pressure is shown in Figure 1.

Fig 1. Maintenance of normal blood pressure

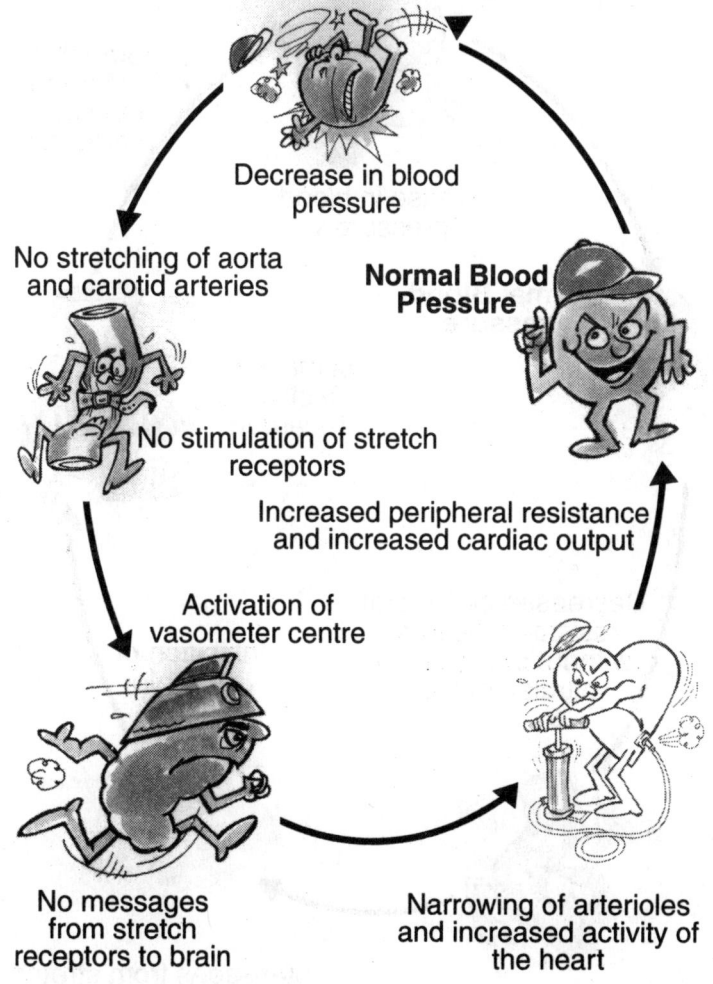

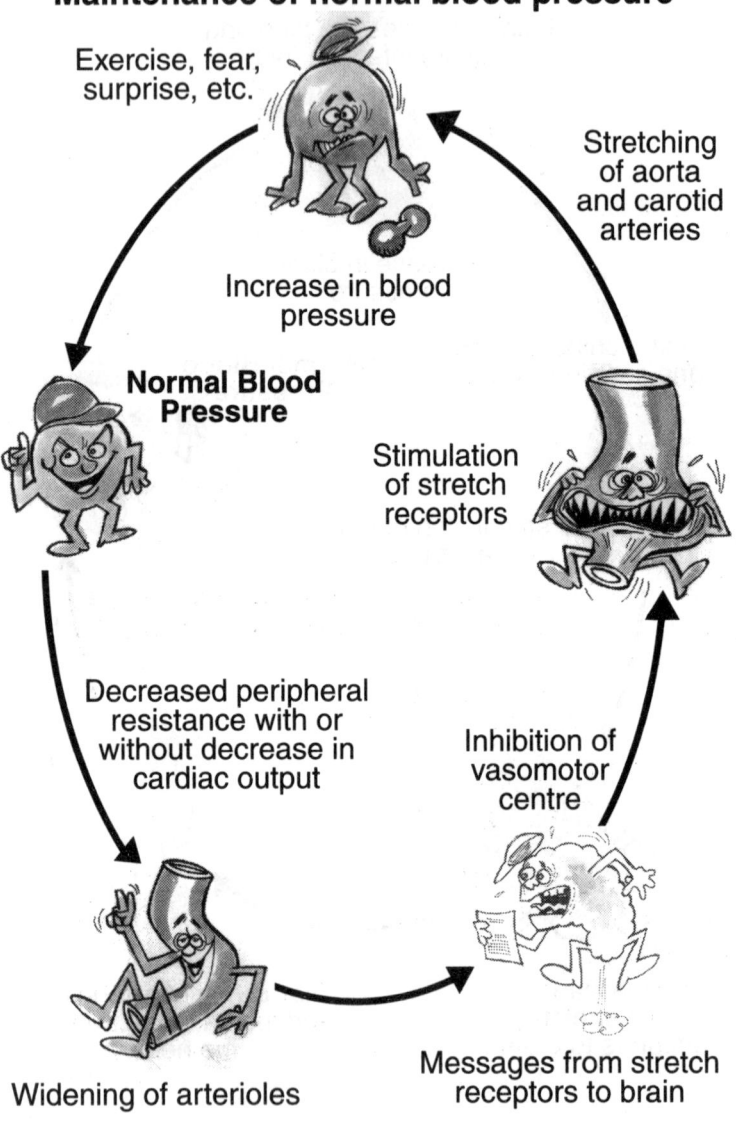

What is hypertension?

Hypertension in adults means

- *persistent systolic pressure* of 140 mm of Hg or more or
- a *persistent diastolic pressure* of 90 mm of Hg or more. Until recently, systolic pressure more than 160 mm of Hg was defined as hypertension. This year, the World Health Organization has recommended that a persistent systolic pressure between 140 and 160 mm of Hg should also be considered as hypertension.

Severity of hypertension is usually expressed on the basis of diastolic pressure as shown in Figure 2. Isolated systolic hypertension is the term used for normal diastolic pressure and systolic pressure above 140 mm of Hg.

If your blood pressure is normal sometimes and high at other times, you may have *"labile hypertension"*. A doctor may then need to record your blood pressure many times before confirming whether you have hypertension or not. In such cases, *it is important for you to cooperate with the doctor and go for regular check-ups.*

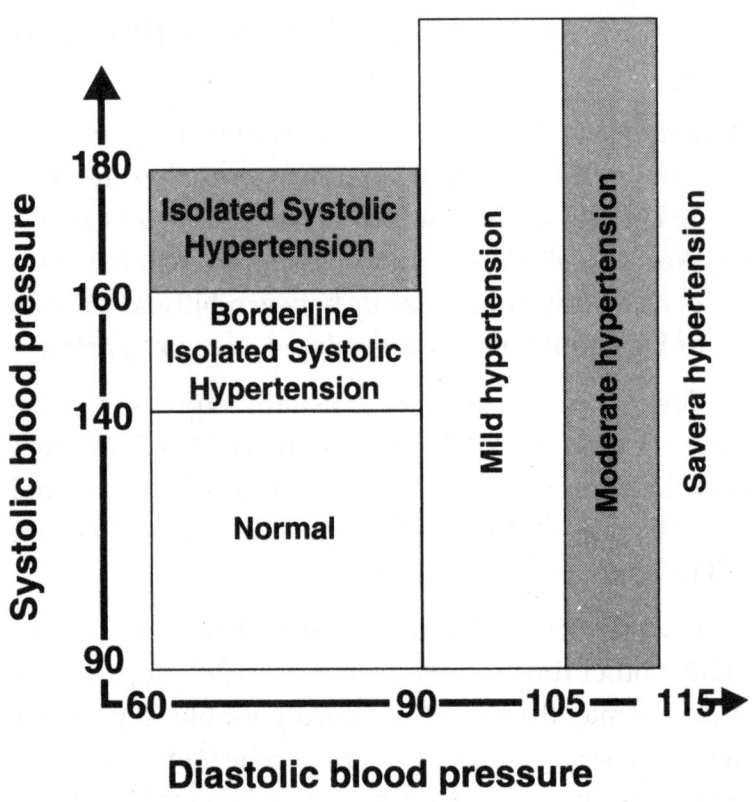

Fig 2. Classification of hypertension

How common is hypertension?

About twenty to thirty percent adults in the urban areas and ten to fifteen percent adults in the rural areas of India have hypertension. These figures are based on hypertension defined as blood pressure more than 140/90 mm of Hg.

High blood pressure is usually detected between thirty-five and fifty-five years of age. *Men and women are at the same risk of developing hypertension. The associated complications of high blood pressure are observed more frequently among men than women.*

What are the causes of hypertension?

Increase in cardiac output or peripheral resistance or both result in hypertension. The exact cause of hypertension in most people cannot be identified. If the cause is not known, the hypertension is called *"primary or essential hypertension"*. The reasons for it include:

- *Stress.* Stress stimulates the brain to release large amounts of the hormones — *"catecholamines"*. These hormones lead to
    - increased cardiac output,
    - increased peripheral resistance,
    - decreased loss of fluid and salt through the kidneys and
    - thickening of the vessel wall.
- *Excessive salt (sodium chloride) in the diet.* Excessive salt increases the blood volume and therefore cardiac output. In addition, excessive salt intake indirectly increases the release of catecholamines.
- *Stiffening and thickening of the walls of the arteries and arterioles.* These changes may be initiated by *hereditary factors*. Aging, diabetes, high cholesterol

and smoking worsen these changes in the arteries. Stiffening of the walls of the arteries reduces their elasticity and results in high systolic pressure. Thickening of the walls of the arterioles increases peripheral resistance and results in high diastolic pressure.

- *Increased retention of water and salt by the kidneys.* This may be due to hereditary factors. Increase in water and salt in body increases blood volume which in turn increases cardiac output.

- *Obesity.* Obesity increases secretion of insulin, a hormone that regulates blood sugar. Insulin may cause thickening of blood vessels and therefore an increase in peripheral resistance. In obese people, the distribution of body fat is also important. A higher waist to hip ratio is more frequently associated with hypertension.

In about five percent of the people with hypertension the exact cause can be identified. When the cause is known, hypertension is called *"secondary hypertension"*. If you are likely to have secondary hypertension, your doctor will suggest many tests. It may take several days to several weeks before you are able to complete all the tests and get their reports. It is important for you to have a positive attitude to deal with the inconvenience and anxiety associated with undergoing several tests. The probable mechanism of primary hypertension is summarised in Figure 3.

Some important causes of secondary hypertension are:

- Diseases of the kidneys and endocrine glands — especially the adrenal glands.
- Long-standing diabetes mellitus.
- Long-term use of oral contraceptives containing oestrogen.
- Use of steroids for many years. (Steroids are a group of drugs commonly used for treatment of asthma, some skin disorders, etc.).
- In-born defects of the *aorta*.
- Pregnancy related, especially during the last three months of pregnancy or immediately after delivery.

Fig 3. Probable mechanisms of primary hypertension

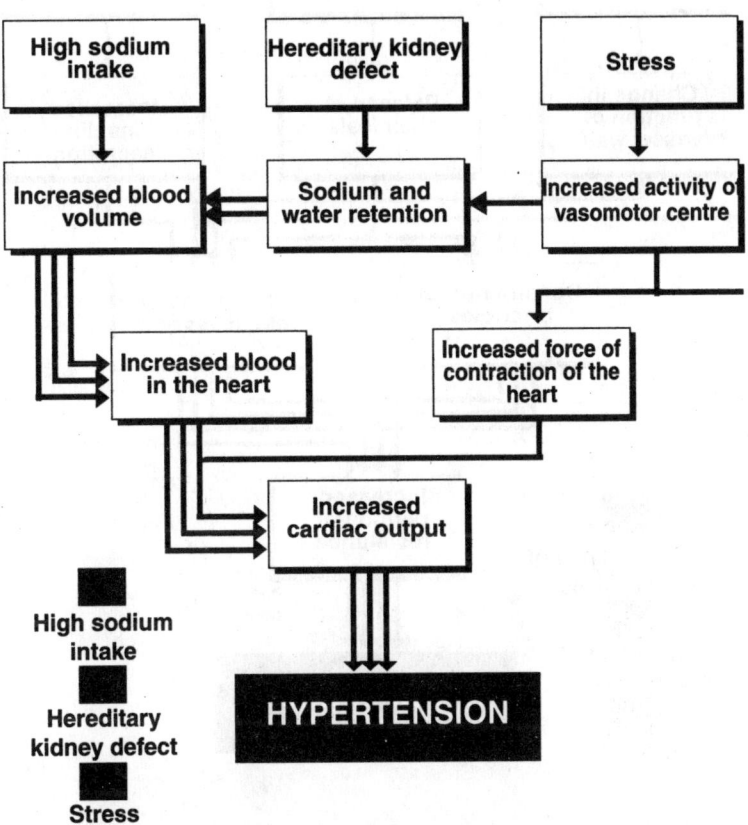

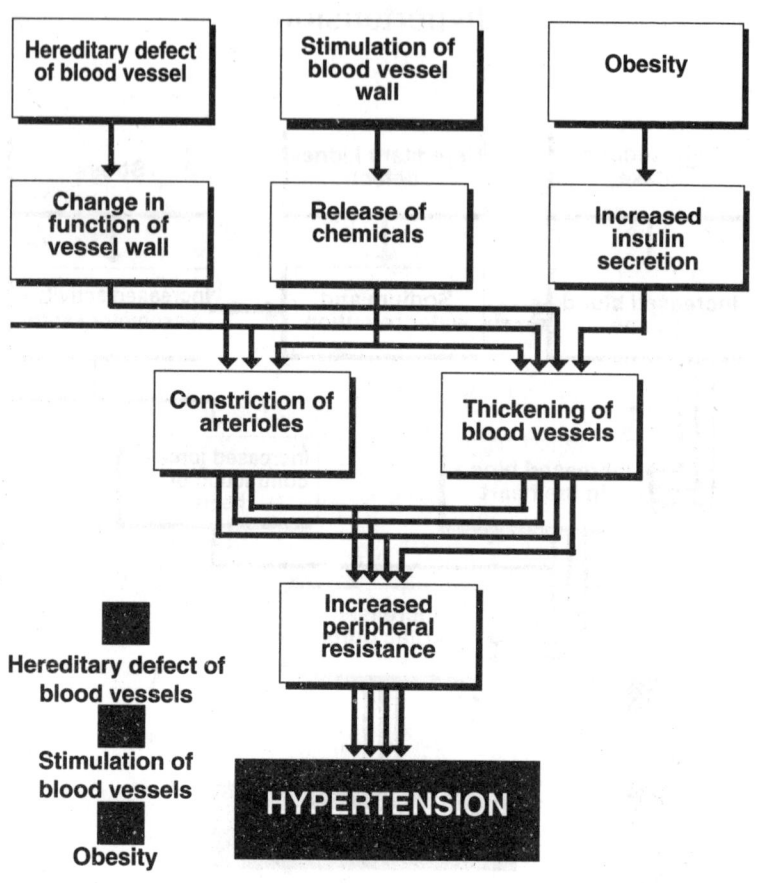

What are the symptoms of hypertension?

Hypertension without complications usually does not cause any symptoms. Thus, you may have high blood pressure for many years before it is detected. It is therefore necessary for you to check your blood pressure as a routine, particularly after the age of thirty years. This will help detection of hypertension as early as possible.

Usually high blood pressure is detected when you visit a doctor for a general check-up or for treatment of some other unrelated disease. Some people with hypertension have headache, dizziness, weakness or merely a feeling of being unwell. High blood pressure is sometimes detected when it leads to serious complications requiring admission to a hospital.

What are the risks and complications associated with hypertension?

High blood pressure by itself can lead to complications such as excessive breathlessness (heart failure), bleeding in the brain (stroke), swelling of the nerves of the eyes (blurred vision) and a tear in the wall of the aorta (aortic dissection). *Such complications develop in about half the people with untreated hypertension over ten years.*

Hypertension also has some indirect effects. These include reduced blood supply to the heart, the kidneys and the lower limbs. This can lead to heart attacks, kidney failure and severe pain in the legs on walking respectively. These complications occur in about thirty percent of people with untreated hypertension over ten years.

Even mild hypertension has a higher risk of heart diseases and strokes. Higher the blood pressure, greater are the risks. Earlier, a high diastolic pressure was considered an important indicator of complications associated with hypertension. Of late, it has been observed that even high systolic pressure is associated with equal, if not more, complications.

Emergency in hypertension

A rapid or sudden increase in the blood pressure to very high levels (usually 240/140 mm of Hg or more) frequently leads to severe headache, blurring of vision, drowsiness, vomiting or breathlessness. This condition called **Malignant Hypertension** *requires emergency treatment at a hospital. This is observed in about one percent of the people with hypertension.*

Hypertension is one among several risk factors for heart attack and strokes. The other risk factors are diabetes, smoking, high cholesterol, older age, males, and heart attacks in the family. Thus, the likelihood of complications occurring in a person with hypertension also depends on the presence or absence of other risk factors. For example, in elderly people with hypertension and a previous heart attack, the risk of a further serious complication is three to five percent every year. On the other hand, in young people with hypertension and without other risk factors, the risk of a further serious complication is only 0.1 percent every year. *It is important to note that in people with hypertension, other risk factors for heart attacks and strokes should also be identified and effectively managed. This will greatly reduce the risks and complications associated with hypertension.*

Which are the risk groups for developing primary hypertension?

- A person with sedentary lifestyle is at twenty to fifty percent greater risk of developing hypertension.
- An overweight person is at two to six times higher risk of developing hypertension.
- If one parent has hypertension, the children are at thirty percent greater risk of developing hypertension.

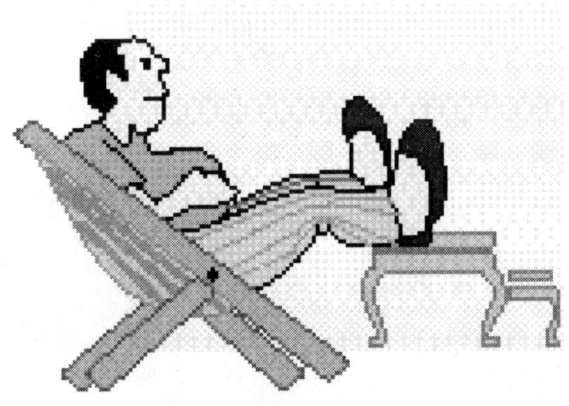

- If both the parents have hypertension, the children are at forty percent more risk of developing hypertension.
- People who are *sensitive to salt intake* are at risk of developing hypertension if they take more than five to six grams of salt per day.

What are the laboratory tests for diagnosis of hypertension?

Your doctor can diagnose hypertension only on the basis of blood pressure values. Some routine tests, however, will be necessary to determine the damage caused by hypertension to important organs and to identify associated conditions that can increase this damage. Special tests will be required if you are suspected to have secondary hypertension. The routine tests normally required are:

- *Blood tests* to identify diabetes, high cholesterol levels and defects in kidney function.
- *Urine tests* to detect diabetes and damage to the kidneys.
- *ECG (Electrocardiogram)* to detect changes in the heart.
- *Chest X-ray* to identify enlargement of the heart or the *aorta*.

How is hypertension controlled?

You can control hypertension by
- changes in lifestyle and/or
- medicines.

Changes in the lifestyle are important for controlling hypertension of any severity. You can reduce systolic pressure by more than 10 mm of Hg and diastolic pressure by more than 7.5 mm of Hg through changes in the lifestyle alone. You can observe the maximum effect from such changes in about three to six months. It is important that you should maintain these changes throughout life for effective control of hypertension.

The **Lifestyle** changes recommended for control of hypertension are:

- *Weight reduction,* especially if you are obese. Nearly two-thirds of overweight people with mild hypertension can control their blood pressure by loosing about fifty percent of the excess weight. You should not lose more than half to one kilogram weight per week. It may be difficult to sustain a more rapid weight loss.

Guidelines for salt intake in hypertension

- You should not take more than five to six grams of salt per day.

- The usual home cooked in urban areas provides about five to six grams salt per day. This is true only if fresh foods are used for cooking.

- If no salt is added while cooking, it provides about two to three grams of salt per day. A person with hypertension can add about half a teaspoon of salt per day. This is true only if processed foods, preserved foods with baking soda are not consumed.

- Use low sodium salts if you want a more salty tastes of food. These are available under various brand names.

- Avoid or at least minimize intake of fast foods as they have a high sodium content.

- Eat natural foods as they contain less sodium. Avoid processed foods they contain more sodium. Avoid pickles and bakery products as they also contain large quantities of salt.

Your blood pressure will fall by about 1.5 mm of Hg for every kilogram of weight loss. You can observe the effect of weight loss on the blood pressure only after losing about four kilos of weight. After a certain level of weight loss, there will be no corresponding decrease in the blood pressure levels.

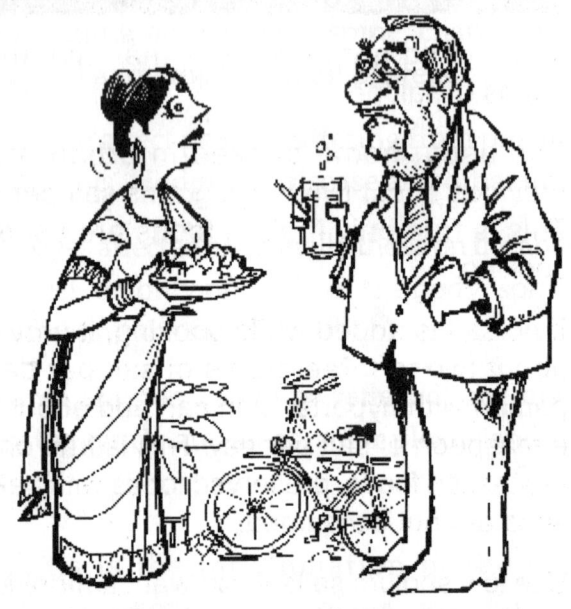

I am taking so many medicines, why is my blood pressure still high?

Weight reduction has other benefits also. It reduces blood cholesterol, risk of heart attacks, backache, pain in the knee joints, etc. It may also prevent diabetes and breast cancer. Weight reduction has no harmful effects.

- *Dietary salt (sodium chloride).* Restriction of salt in diet is effective in about sixty percent of people with hypertension. The response is especially better in elderly people.

- *Regular exercises.* Walking, running, swimming, aerobics, games and cycling reduce blood pressure by 5-10 mm of Hg. About thirty to sixty minutes of walking three to five times a week is a good exercise for control of hypertension. You should avoid exercises such as weight lifting as they increase blood pressure. It is necessary to take advice from your doctor before starting any exercise programme.

- *Alcohol intake.* You should not take more than sixty millilitres (ml) of whisky neat (without adding soda or water), two hundred and forty ml of wine, or seven hundred and twenty ml of beer per day. Your blood pressure will rise to abnormal levels if you take larger quantities. Similarly, your blood pressure will come down if you reduce high alcohol intake.

- *Relaxation techniques.* Several studies have indicated that regular yoga, meditation and reducing mental stress help control hypertension. These methods probably increase the tolerance to psychological stress. You will be able to see the effect of relaxation techniques after about eight weeks of regular practice.

It is important to note that additional lifestyle changes are necessary if other risk factors such as diabetes, smoking, and high cholesterol are present.

Medicines are required for control of hypertension if you belong to one of the following groups:

1. Mild hypertension not controlled by the lifestyle changes followed for three to six months.
2. Moderate hypertension.

3. Severe hypertension.
4. Isolated systolic hypertension of 140-180 mm of Hg not controlled by the lifestyle changes followed for three to six months.
5. Isolated systolic hypertension more than 180 mm of Hg.

Medicines commonly used for controlling high blood pressure include the following groups:

- *ACE (angiotensin converting enzyme) inhibitors.* These medicines control blood pressure by reducing peripheral resistance. Persistent dry cough is a common side effect of ACE inhibitors.
- *Calcium channel blockers.* These medicines mainly reduce peripheral resistance. Some medicines in this group also reduce the cardiac output. Common side effects are abnormal slowing or quickening of heart beat, constipation and swelling of the feet.
- *Beta-blockers.* These medicines mainly reduce cardiac output. Beta blockers are preferred if there is heart disease along with hypertension. Fatigue and depression are two common side effects of beta blockers.
- *Alpha-blockers.* These medicines mainly reduce peripheral resistance. Common side effects are abnormal quickening of heart beat and giddiness on standing up suddenly.
- *Diuretics.* They result in increased salt and water loss from the body. This reduces the cardiac output.

Diuretics also reduce peripheral resistance when taken for a long time. Common side effects are weakness and leg cramps.

The common treatment plan for hypertension is as shown in Figure 4.

Medicines used to control hypertension vary from person to person. The doctor's choice of medicine will

Fig 4. Guidelines for treatment of Hypertension

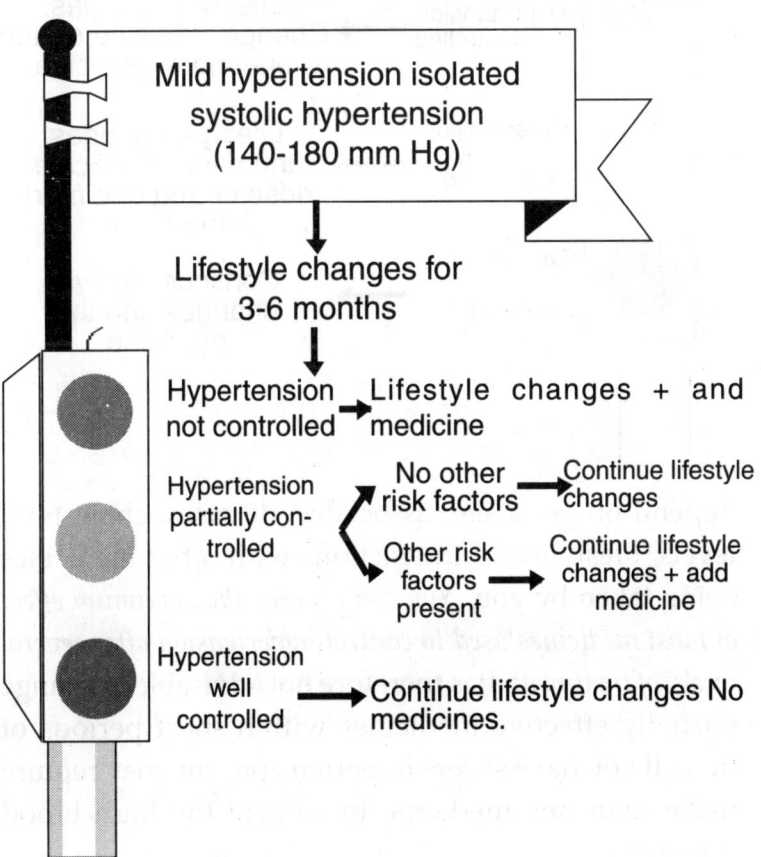

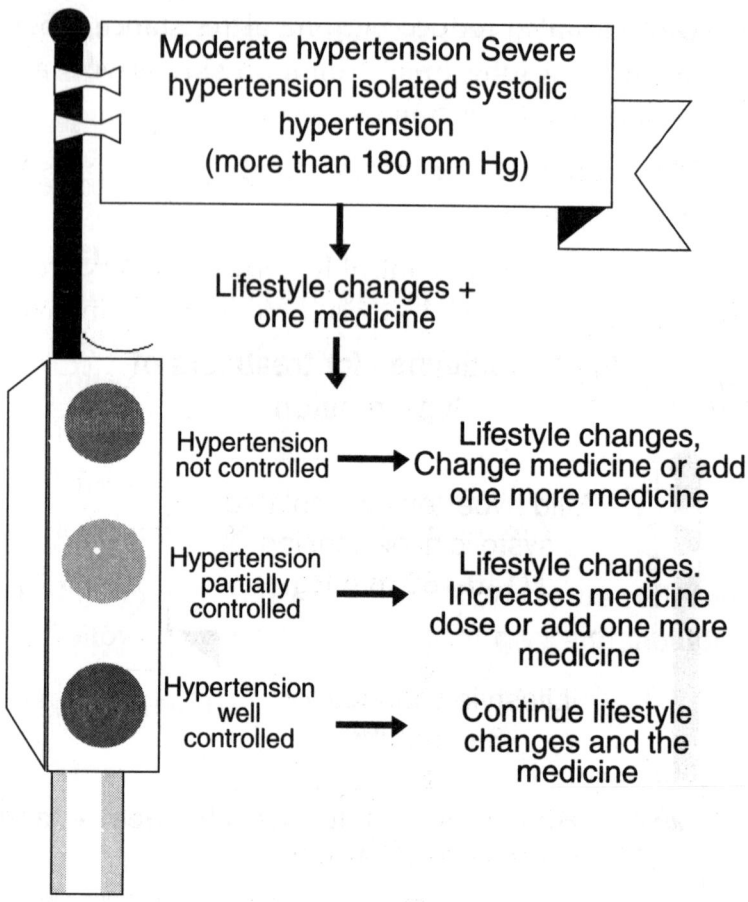

depend on your age, associated diseases, cholesterol levels, lifestyle and interactions with other medicines being taken by you. *You can observe the maximum effect of most medicines used to control hypertension after several weeks of treatment.* It is therefore not advisable to change partially effective medicines within short periods of time. If you have severe hypertension, you may require more than one medicine to control the high blood pressure.

Some pain killers interfere with the effect of medicines used to control high blood pressure. You should consult your doctor before taking any other medicines.

The management of other risk factors such as diabetes, high cholesterol and smoking is very important in people with hypertension.

Benefits of quitting smoking

When you quit smoking, the body begins to recover within twenty minutes.

- *After twenty minutes:* Your blood pressure drops and pulse rate drops to normal.
- *After eight hours:* Carbon monoxide level in the blood drops to normal. Oxygen level in blood increases to normal.
- *After twenty-four hours:* Chance of a heart attack decreases.
- *After forty-eight hours:* Ability to smell and taste is enhanced.
- *Between two weeks to three weeks*: Blood circulation improves. You can walk more easily. Lung functions increase up to thirty percent.
- *Between one to nine months:* Cough, congestion of the nose, fatigue and breathlessness decrease. Hair-like projections in the lungs grow and therefore dust, bacteria, etc. are removed more efficiently.
- *After one year*: Excess risk of coronary heart disease is half that of a smoker.

- *After five years:* Lung cancer death rate decreases by almost half. Stroke risk is reduced to that of nonsmoker five to fifteen years after quitting. Risk of cancer of the mouth, throat and food-pipe reduces to half of smoker's risk.
- *After ten years:* Lung cancer death rate is similar to that of a nonsmoker. Risk of cancer of the mouth, throat, food-pipe, bladder and kidneys decreases.
- *After fifteen years:* Risk of heart diseases is that of a nonsmoker.

Source: Center for Disease Control and American Cancer Society

How long should the medicines be taken?

You may have to take medicines for the control of hypertension throughout life. In rare cases when the cause of high blood pressure is identified and cured, you can stop taking medicines.

Reducing or stopping medicines for up to four years may be possible in about one-third of the people with hypertension after good control of blood pressure. *It is important to note that this decision has to be taken only by your doctor because there can be a rise in the blood pressure after reducing or stopping medicines.* A rise in the blood pressure during this period can be treated as soon as possible if you go for regular check-ups.

Sometimes the blood pressure falls below normal levels while taking medicines. Fall in blood pressure may cause giddiness, weakness, and rarely fainting. Regular check-up is therefore necessary to modify the treatment. The frequency of check-up should be as advised by your doctor.

Sometimes people take more medicines if they "feel" that they have high blood pressure. Similarly, they take less medicines or stop them if they "feel" that they have low blood pressure. These feelings may not always be true. It is important to check the blood pressure with a sphygmomanometer to find out the correct blood pressure. You should consult a doctor whenever you "feel" that your blood pressure levels are either higher or lower than normal.

Are special diets recommended for control of hypertension?

The only reliable dietary modification for control of hypertension is reduced intake of sodium salts. Some studies have suggested that diets containing large quantities of potassium, calcium or magnesium reduce blood pressure. Diets rich in potassium may have their effect on blood pressure by changing the proportion of dietary sodium to dietary potassium. Fresh fruits and vegetables are rich in potassium and fibre.

Some other studies have indicated that changing the type of fat in the diet may reduce blood pressure. *It is important to note that these benefits have not been observed **consistently** in several well designed studies. Therefore, these nutrition supplements are not routinely recommended for the control of hypertension.* Vegetarian or high fibre diets may reduce high blood pressure but this needs further investigation.

How can hypertension be prevented?

Hypertension may be prevented by adopting the following lifestyle changes:
- weight reduction in obese people;
- reduction of salt intake in those who take more than six grams salt per day;
- reduction in alcohol intake in those who take more than the quantity mentioned earlier;
- exercise for those with sedentary lifestyle.

These lifestyle changes are more important for people who have diastolic pressure between 85-89 mm of Hg. People with this range of diastolic pressure are at two times greater risk of developing hypertension at a later stage.

Studies have not convincingly indicated that reducing stress, supplementation of potassium, calcium, magnesium or fish oil and high-fibre diet prevent hypertension. A high-fibre diet has other health benefits. It reduces cholesterol and cancer of the intestine.

Risks of hypertension

Untreated hypertension increases the risk of:

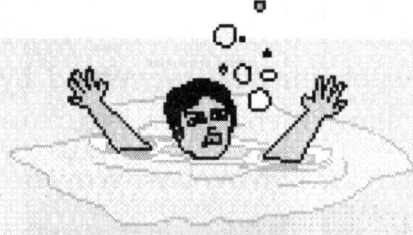

- heart attacks by two to three times
- strokes by two to four times
- death by two times

Untreated hypertension decreases life span by about ten to twenty years

Benefits of treatment of hypertension

If decrease in diastolic pressure by 5-6 mm of Hg and systolic pressure by 10-14 mm of Hg is maintained for about five years there is:

- decrease in risk of stroke by thirty eight percent;
- decrease in risk of heart disease by sixteen percent
- decrease in risk of death by twenty one percent

Benefits of decrease in high blood pressure are observed by about two to three years after treatment

What are the current research areas for the management of hypertension?

1. Several groups of medicines are being tested for more effective control of hypertension with lesser side effects. These include Renin inhibitors, Angiotensin II receptor antagonist, Endopep-tidase inhibitors and Endothelin antagonists.
2. Research is needed to identify those people who are sure to develop hypertension at a later stage. Lifestyle changes can then be applied specifically to these people to prevent hypertension.
3. *Aspirin* reduces risks of second and subsequent heart attacks and strokes. Research studies are required to find out if aspirin can reduce the risks of a first heart attack or a first stroke in people with hypertension.
4. *Echocardiography,* an ultrasound examination of the heart has shown that hypertension associated with thickening of the heart muscle and increased weight of the heart is an early warning of heart

problems. Most drugs used for the management of hypertension reverse these changes in the heart. Research studies are underway to identify whether this reversal reduces the risks of heart problems associated with hypertension.

What is the desirable family support for a person with hypertension?

Family members can help to reduce stressful situations within the family which is an important cause of high blood pressure. Support of the family members is also important for the following reasons:

1. A person with hypertension needs to make long term adjustments in his/her lifestyle.
2. Long-term regular treatment with medicines is usually required.
3. The regularity and continuity of taking medicines requires active involvement of the family members.
4. Fear of risks associated with hypertension may itself lead to stressful situations.
5. Some people worry about the risks associated with hypertension. They do not readily accept that regular treatment reduces risks associated with hypertension.

AYURVEDA

The ancient scriptures or Ayurveda do not have any detailed description of hypertension and its management. High blood pressure is described as one of the complications and causes of heart diseases. Practitioners of Ayurveda believe that hypertension was not a major health problem in the past mainly because the lifestyle in those times caused very little stress.

What are the causes of hypertension?

According to Ayurveda, heart is the seat of consciousness. Emotions directly affect the heart and heart diseases occur when these emotions cause unhappiness.

Hypertension results when there are imbalances in the body *"humors"* due to physical or emotional trauma. These imbalances can also be due to hereditary factors, diet and lifestyle which do not maintain the balance in the humours, accumulation of fat in the body, stress, old age and anxiety.

What is the treatment for hypertension?

Ayurveda lays special emphasis on control of hypertension through changes in the lifestyle. It strongly recommends meditation for maintaining harmony between body and the mind. This harmony reduces stress and helps to sustain a relaxed mind. Relaxation of mind leads to behavioural changes in a person with hypertension. These changes in behaviour and attitude help reduce adverse reactions to stressful situations. Ability to control temper and keeping calm under all circumstances checks high blood pressure. *"Yogasans, Yoganidra* and *Pranayama"* are also very effective in controlling high blood pressure.

Certain liquids such as coconut water and lime juice and wearing *"rudraksha beads"* are believed to reduce *pitta* and relax the mind and body. The combination of reduced pitta and relaxed mind control hypertension.

Salt restriction is one of the important factors in control of hypertension in the Ayurvedic system also. The guidelines for salt restriction are the same as those listed in the section on Allopathy.

The Ayurvedic medicines recommended for treatment of primary hypertension are:

- *Gokshruad and Guggul.* These medicines are derived from Gokhru herb. They increase the loss of salt and water from the body. This reduces the volume of blood and therefore cardiac output. Guggul also maintains elasticity of the blood vessels.

- *Sarpagandha.* This is a product of Rauwolfia Serpentina, a herb effective for the control of high blood pressure. This medicine reduces cardiac output. Long term use of Sarpagandha, especially in excess dose, has *adverse* effects.

  Some studies have indicated that the combination of Rauwolfia Serpentina, Abhal and Corn-Silk controls primary hypertension. This combination reduces peripheral resistance and cardiac output. This medicine is generally used in Unani system of medicine, which is similar to Ayurveda.

- *Punarnava.* This plant extract increases loss of salt and water from the body. The cardiac output therefore decreases.

- *Akeek Pisti.* This medicine improves tone of the muscles of the heart. It is believed to reduce cardiac output.

The management of secondary hypertension requires additional treatment.

How long should the medicines be taken?

According to the Ayurveda, early and mild hypertension can be effectively controlled by changes in the lifestyle. Some people may require medicines for a few weeks to few months. Medicines are required throughout life to control severe hypertension, especially if there is damage to organs such as heart, kidneys and the eyes.

> **?**
>
> **DO YOU KNOW THAT**
>
> It is not necessary for a person with hypertension to **suffer** from hypertension

HOMOEOPATHY

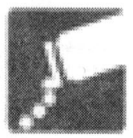

The definition, risks and complications of hypertension described in Homoeopathy are the same as in Allopathy. The difference between the two systems is in *Individualization*. Homoeopathic medicines for hypertension, just as in all other diseases, vary from person to person. A Homoeopathy doctor attempts to identify hypertensive personality — people who are likely to develop hypertension. Stress is considered to be one of the main causes of hypertension. There are several people who have emotional and physical stress. Of these, some have normal blood pressure, some develop labile hypertension and some have high blood pressure. The Homoeopathic system identifies personality traits that can lead to hypertension. Most common among these traits are: aggressive, irritable or introvert people, irregular or sedentary lifestyle, obese people, and anxious or worried state of the mind. Apart from these common factors, severe hypertension secondary to chronic disease or inflammation of the kidney, damage to the kidney due to stones or diabetes and certain tumours around the kidney also cause hypertension.

Homoeopathic medicines offer support to the body's natural capacity to prevent and cure diseases very quickly and permanently. The treatment includes identifying behavioural symptoms in a person and prescribing medicines for those symptoms. These medicines affect the controlling mechanism of the mind on the body. By identifying early defects in the functions of the body, Homoeopathic medicines are able to prevent damage to the structure of the body tissues and organs. Diseases are usually detected when there are structural changes in the body.

What are the early signs of hypertension?

Factors leading to hypertension are:
- increased irritability and tendency to become angry or violent;
- very busy people working under stressful conditions;
- lack of sleep;
- headaches, especially throbbing pain, which is associated with anger and working under stress;
- dizziness;
- flushed face on exertion;
- excessive craving for salt;
- obesity;
- and sudden emotional shock.

You and your doctor

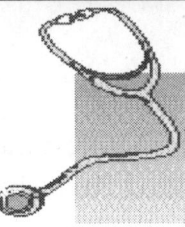

- Your doctor is the best person to choose the type of drug(s) required to control your hypertension

- The doctor may need to change medicines or use a combination of medicines to suit your specific requirements.

- It is important for you to cooperate with the doctor for monitoring of the blood pressure when treatment is started or when it is modified.

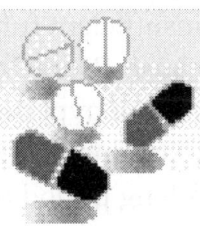

What are the stages of hypertension?

Homoeopathy identifies three stages of manifestations of hypertension. These stages are classified on the basis of susceptibility to diseases acquired by the body. This susceptibility, which is reflected in predisposing factors of a disease and causes long-term illnesses, is called *Miasm*.

1. ***Hypertension due to Psora Miasm.*** Deficiency or insufficient functions of human tissues and organs cause Psora Miasm. The common causes of this type of hypertension are mental and physical stress. Excitement, anger, anxiety, worries or tension over a long period of time are the main causes of stress.

2. ***Hypertension due to Sycosis Miasm.*** Excess or increased function of human tissues and organs cause Sycosis Miasm. The common causes of this type of hypertension are metabolic changes due to abnormalities or diseases in other organs in the body. For example, diabetes, some diseases of the kidney, thickening of the blood vessels and use of contraceptive drugs can result in hypertension due to Sycosis Miasm.

3. ***Hypertension due to Syphilitic Miasm.*** Changes in, or abnormal function of, human tissues and organs are causes of Syphilitic Miasm. In this type of hypertension, there is widespread damage to organs such as heart, kidney, eyes and the brain.

What is the treatment for hypertension?

The goal of the treatment of hypertension with Homoeopathic medicines is not just to lower the blood pressure but also to completely destroy the disease process. A Homoeopathic doctor will ask you many questions, some of which you may *feel* are not related to your health problems. The doctor will assess all your symptoms in detail and determine the stage of your disease. Broadly, the doctor will place you in any one of the following groups of changes in you organs and tissues:

- *Functional change*. In this group there is no damage to the structure of either blood vessels or other organs of the body. There are early changes in the function of tissues and organs which are normally not detected by any laboratory investigations. At this stage of the disease there may not be any specific symptoms of hypertension. Homoeopathic medicines are required for about four to six weeks at this stage of hypertension.

- *Reversible structural change.* In this group there are early changes in the structure of blood vessels and other organs such as adrenal glands, kidneys,

Common misconceptions about hypertension.

- *Hypertension is commonly called blood pressure.* This is not correct. Every person has blood pressure because it is necessary for the flow of blood in the body. Hypertension means high blood pressure.

- *If blood pressure reading by two doctors are different on the same day, it means that one of the instruments is not accurate.* This is not always correct. Two doctors may record different levels of your blood pressure because of its normal variations during the day.

- *Smoking and drinking coffee are cause of hypertension.* This has not been observed in several well-designed studies in Allopathy. Smoking and drinking two to three cups of coffee increase blood pressure temporarily. They do not lead to persistent high blood pressure. A person who drinks coffee regularly will not have any increase in blood pressure due to coffee.

- *Hard work causes stress and, therefore, hypertension.* This is not always correct. Work done with a relaxed mind, without hurry, without the pressure of meeting deadlines, and without losing temper does not lead to stress. It, therefore, does not lead to hypertension.

heart, etc. A person in this group may complain of headache, giddiness, restlessness, or tiredness. These symptoms could be due to hypertension. The Homoeopathic medicines for treatment of this stage should be continued for at least two to three months. Some people may require longer treatment. A practitioner of Homoeopathy believes that this stage of hypertension can be cured with medicines.

- *Irreversible structural change.* In this group there are chances of irreversible changes in the blood vessels, heart, kidneys, eyes, brain, etc. At this stage the disease cannot be cured. Medicines are prescribed to avoid complications and prevent further damage to the tissues and organs of the body.

The Homoeopathic medicines for the treatment of hypertension act through the brain and decrease either cardiac output or peripheral resistance or both. Treatment with Homoeopathic medicines is usually reviewed every two weeks because the medicines result in rapid changes in the functions of the tissues and organs of the body. It is therefore important to change either the medicine or the dose to suit the individual requirements. Most people start feeling better after the first few doses itself. However, complete cure takes time and therefore long-term treatment is necessary.

There may be mild and temporary side effects of taking Homoeopathic medicines. These medicines, like all other medicines, should not be stopped suddenly as they may result in undesirable effects. The lifestyle changes recommended in the Homoeopathic system are the same as those detailed in the section on Allopathy.

NATURE CURE

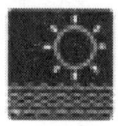

The aim of Nature Cure is to remove the basic cause of disease through appropriate use of natural elements. It is not just a system of healing but also a way of life.

A practitioner of Nature Cure believes that early symptoms suggesting high blood pressure should not be ignored. These early symptoms include dizziness, aches, pain in the heart region, frequent passing of urine, tiredness, irritability, emotional upset and sometimes lack of sleep and appetite.

What is the treatment for hypertension?

Nature Cure recommends hydrotherapy (treatment with water), mud therapy, diet therapy, and relaxation for control of hypertension.

- *Hydrotherapy* increases circulation of blood to the skin surface. It also restores elasticity of the arterioles and the capillaries. Hydrotherapy includes:
- *Full wet sheet pack.* In this treatment, body is wrapped in wet sheet, dry sheet and a blanket, in that order, for one hour. Full wet sheet pack decreases peripheral resistance.
- *Cold spinal bath.* In this bath, you need to lie down in a special tub. It is important to note that only backbone is kept in contact with water for twenty to thirty minutes. This bath inhibits the vasomotor centre. Thus, the peripheral resistance decreases. Cold spinal bath also relaxes the mind.
- *Neutral half bath.* Sitting in a tub filled with lukewarm water up to waist level for twenty minutes relaxes blood vessels of the legs. This results in lower blood pressure levels. It is important to cover head with a cold cloth during neutral half bath.

- *Chest pack.* Covering chest with cold cloth, dry cloth and a blanket, in that order, for one hour reduces the cardiac output.

- *Ice massage.* Sliding ice cubes on the backbone and head for six to seven minutes reduces activity of the vasomotor centre. Thus the peripheral resistance decreases.

- *Cold hip bath.* In this bath, the waist region is kept in a special tub partially filled with cold water for fifteen to twenty minutes. You should rub the stomach with a soft cloth every few minutes. After this bath, you have to either take a brisk walk or lie down in bed covered with a blanket for fifteen to twenty minutes. Cold hip bath removes "poisons" from the digestive system. It also controls high blood pressure indirectly. A cold wet towel or mud pack can be used instead of the bath.

- *Mud bath.* In this treatment, mud paste is applied to your body and allowed to dry. After about one hour, you should have cold water bath. Mud bath relaxes blood vessels. The peripheral resistance therefore decreases.

- ***Dietary changes*** are important for control of hypertension in Nature Cure. Reduced salt intake is very important. Tender coconut juice, butter milk, coriander seeds decoction and barley water increase loss of salt from the body. They are therefore important for control of hypertension. Drinking eight to ten glasses of water per day also removes salt from the body. Other dietary changes recommended in Nature Cure are:

- *Fresh fruits.* A traditional diet should be replaced by a diet of fresh fruits and vegetables. This diet removes "poisons" from the body and therefore the blood pressure comes down.

    A Nature Cure doctor will recommend an exclusive diet of fresh fruits and vegetables for at least one week. Fruits should be eaten every five hours three times a day. Apples, oranges, mangoes, guava, pineapples and water melon are the best fruits for this diet. Bananas and jack fruit should be avoided.

    After one week of a diet of fruits, you will be advised to take fresh milk. It is important to note that the milk should be boiled only once. Cereals such as rice and wheat are added after two weeks of fruit diet.

- *Vegetables.* Raw vegetables such as cucumber, carrot, tomatoes, onion, radish, cabbage and spinach help reduce high blood pressure. They should be cut into small pieces and seasoned with a pinch of salt and juice of one lemon. Garlic relaxes arterioles and the peripheral resistance therefore decreases. The result is decrease in high blood pressure. Garlic may reduce cardiac output. About two to three capsules of garlic per day help control hypertension.

    Indian gooseberry (amla) is also recommended for people with high blood pressure. One tablespoon each of amla juice and honey should be taken every morning. Lemon juice is also believed to be effective in the control of hypertension.

Watermelon, especially its seeds, relaxes the arterioles resulting in a decrease in peripheral resistance.

High potassium and calcium increase the loss of sodium from the body. This reduces volume of blood and therefore cardiac output. Fruits and vegetables are generally rich in potassium. Milk and milk products are rich sources of calcium.

- *Exercise.* Walking is generally believed to be the best exercise for a person with hypertension. Exercise reduces emotional stress, activates the muscles and therefore improves the blood circulation. After the high blood pressure returns to normal levels, exercises such as cycling, swimming and jogging are recommended.

- *Yoga therapy.* Regular practice of Yogasanas, deep breathing and meditation help to reduce the blood pressure by reducing stress. Some yogasanas should not be done if you have severe hypertension.

- *Rest.* It is important for a person with hypertension to have restful sleep for about eight hours every night. Rest reduces stress by relaxing the mind and the body. Decrease in stress over a period of time leads to maintenance of normal blood pressure.

Natural treatment for hypertension

- **Hydrotherapy**
- **Cold spinal bath**
- **Neutral half bath**
- **Chest pack**
- **Ice massage**
- **Cold hip bath**
- **Mud bath**
- **Dietary changes**
- **Fresh fruits**
- **Vegetables**
- **Exercise**
- **Yoga therapy**
- **Rest**

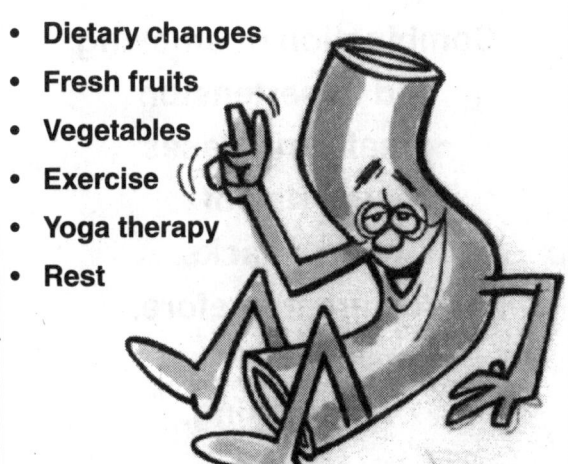

HEALTH TIP

Combination of smoking
and hypertension
greatly increases
the risk of
heart attacks.
You are, therefore,
advised to give
up smoking.

Definitions

Aorta is the largest artery of the body that emerges from the heart.

Arteries are the blood vessels that carry blood from the heart to various parts of the body.

Arterioles are the smallest branches of the arteries. They largely determine the peripheral resistance.

Capillaries are a network of small blood vessels through which oxygen and nutrients are supplied to various parts of the body.

Cardiac output is the volume of blood pumped by the heart per minute. It is usually five litres per minute.

Carotid arteries supply blood to the neck and the head including the brain.

Cholesterol is a type of body fat that can be measured in the blood. High cholesterol is one important cause of heart attacks.

Endocrine glands secrete hormones directly into the blood stream.

Hereditary factors are factors that are transmitted from one generation to the other.

Hormones are chemical substances produced by specific organs having effects on other organs of the body.

Obesity is more than twenty percent of normal weight for age, height and sex of a person.

Peripheral resistance is the resistance to blood flow through the arterial system. This resistance is mainly in the arterioles.

Pitta is heat and energy in body. It is responsible for the process of digestion. It is responsible for all chemical and metabolic changes in the body.

Stroke is a condition where either there is rupture or obstruction of a blood vessel of the brain. This may lead to sudden paralysis and/or decrease or loss of consciousness.

Vasomotor centre is a group of nerve cells situated in the brain. It helps in maintaining normal blood pressure.

Veins are blood vessels that carry blood from various parts of the body to the heart.

References

Allopathy

Braunwald E. (ed.). *Heart disease: A text book of cardiovascular medicine.* 1992.

Collins R. et al. Lancet 1990; 335: 827-838.

Laragh J H, Brenner B M. (ed.) *Hypertension - Pathophysiology, diagnosis and management.* 1995.

Macmohan S. et al. *Lancet* 1990; 335: 765-774.

Puddley I B. et al. *Hypertension* 1992; 20: 533-541.

Stamler R. et al. *JAMA* 1989; 262: 1801-1807.

Stamler J. et al. *Archives of Internal Medicine* 1993; 153:598-615

Swodes J D. (ed.) *Text book of hypertension.* 1994.

Trials of hypertension prevention collaborative research group. *JAMA* 1992; 267:1213-1220.

Whelton P K. *Lancet* 1994; 344: 101-106

World Health Organization Technical Report Series. Hypertension control, 862, 1996.

Ayurveda

Sharma Vaid Shri Goberdhan Sharma. *Ashtanghridaya.* 1991; 13, 179, 188-189.

Sharma P V. *Charak Sutrasthan.* 1981; 30/26

Sharma P V. *Dravyaguna Vigyan.* Vol II. 1978; 219,36,630

Homoeopathy

Allen Henry J. *The Chronic Miasms* Vol. I.

Boericke Williams. *Homoeopathic Materia Medica.*

Hahnemann Samuel. *Organon of medicine.*

Kanjilal J N. *Writings on Homoeopathy.*

Kent J T. *Lectures on Homoeopathic Philosophy.*

Mazumdar K P. *Lectures on Homoeopathic Therapeutics.*

Ortega Sanchez Procosco. *Notes on Miasms.*